The Doctor Says:

Let's Talk About Body Safety

Written by

Dr. Pat Morgan

Illustrated by

CJ Hampton

D1294454

The Doctor Says: Let's Talk About Body Safety © 2023 by Dr. Pat Morgan
Illustrations by CJ Hampton
Published by Palm Enterprises, LLC

Printed in the United States of America

ISBN: 979-8-9869716-3-6

This book is dedicated to all children.
You have the power within to be BRAVE!

Writing and completing any book takes persistence, dedication and lots of love and help from those around you. I must acknowledge several people whose advice, guidance, and encouragement have helped me along the way:

My young adult children (Z and C) – I love you more than I can ever say!

Nicholas – for your creative mind!

My "Bellah Bellah" – for always being there!

Dr. Jsahna Simmons – my sister friend & "Creative Consultant."

CJ Hampton – you are an "Illustrator extraordinaire."

Alicia Ingram – for keeping me on task.

SKY– for your attention to detail!

And to all those who read the first draft, my Sister Circle, and all my loved ones for their tremendous support!

Lastly, thank you to the parents and young readers of this book for entrusting me with sharing this important message.

-Dr. Pat

For the Grown-Ups:

BEFORE you read this book with your child or have your child read this book:

If you have your own history of abuse, this book may serve as a trigger. Please protect yourself and always know it is never too late to get help for yourself.

1. You know your child best! Please be prepared to answer questions – during and after reading this book.

2. This book is an introduction for pre-school and primary school-aged children on the topic of keeping their bodies safe.

3. This book teaches empowerment to children in a child-friendly manner. It can be read to a young child by an adult OR the independent reader can read it on their own.

4. Please be sure to see the "**For the Grown-Ups**" section AFTER you read this book, even if you have an independent reader.

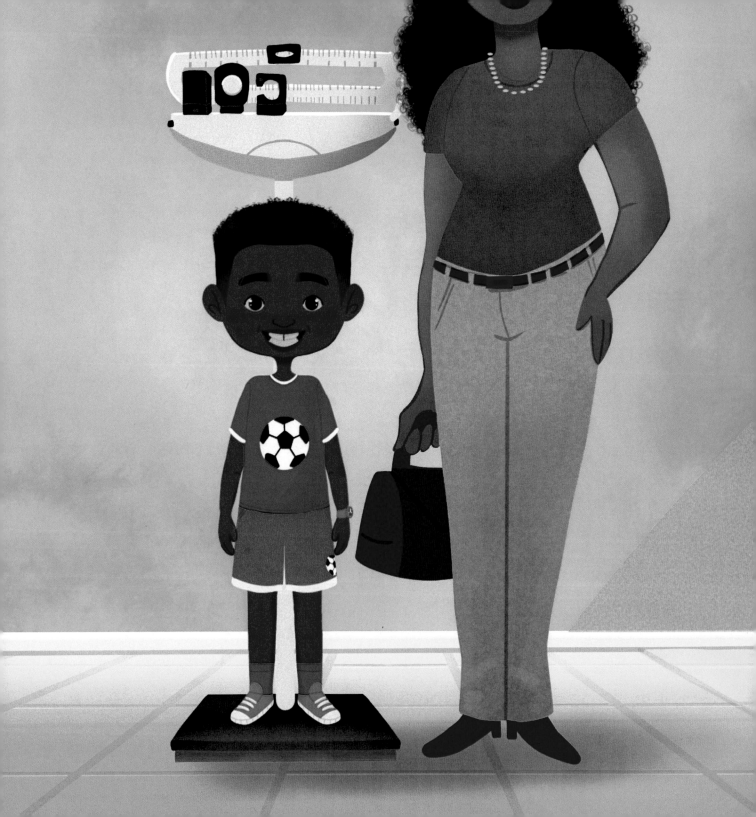

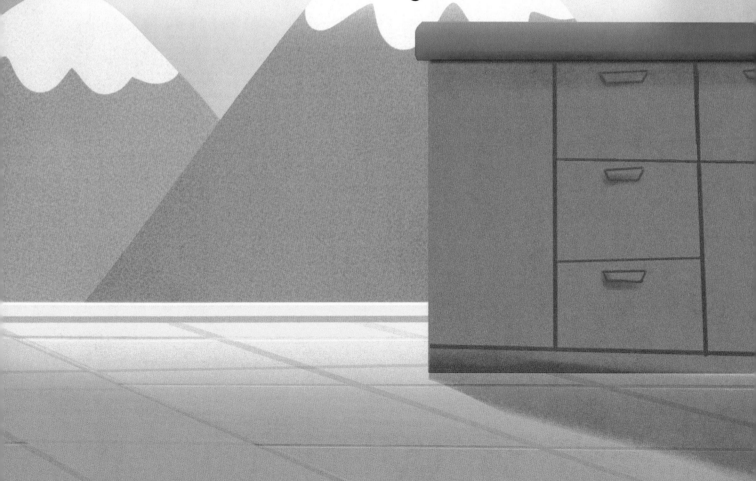

Going to the doctor is really cool.
Sometimes I'm sick and have to miss school.

Most times I'm okay and she tells me so.
She makes sure I'm healthy from head to toe.

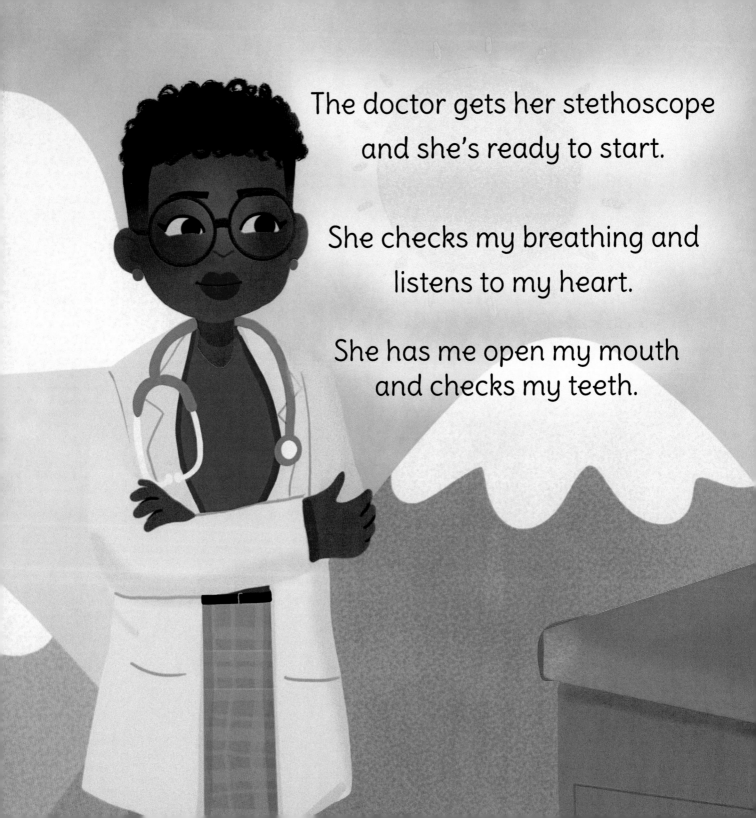

The doctor gets her stethoscope
and she's ready to start.

She checks my breathing and
listens to my heart.

She has me open my mouth
and checks my teeth.

The doctor also feels my belly
and looks at my toes and feet.

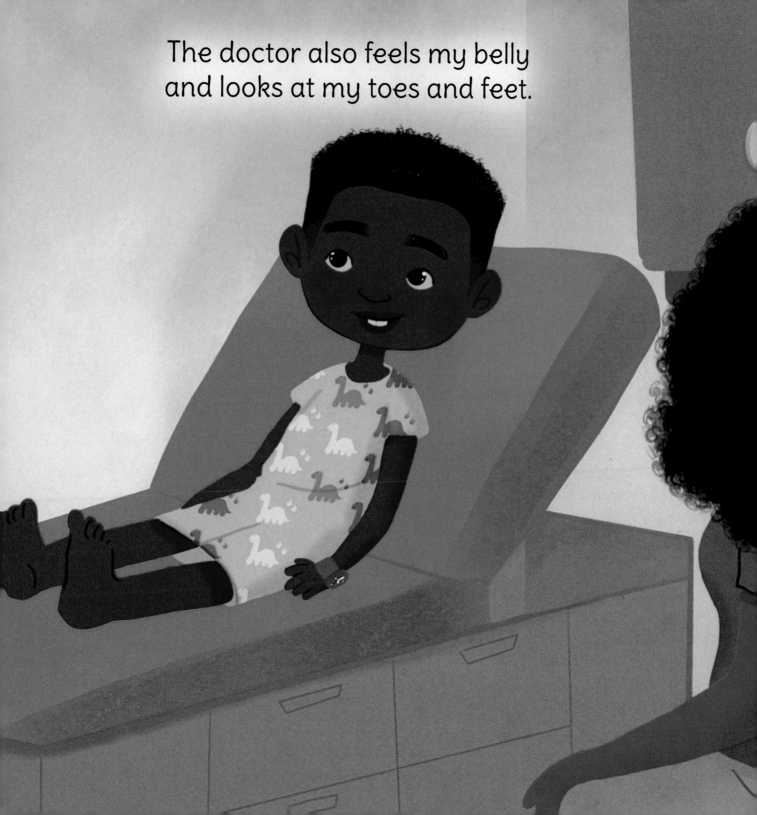

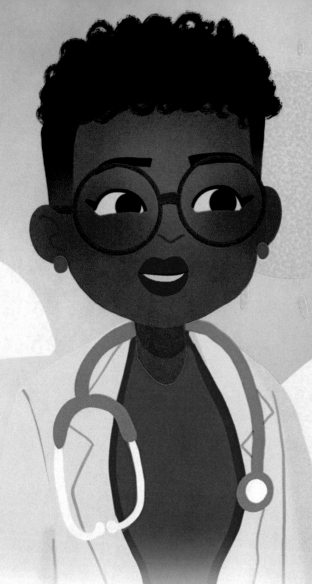

Near the end of the check-up,
the doctor says to me,
"Before we are done, let's talk about body safety."

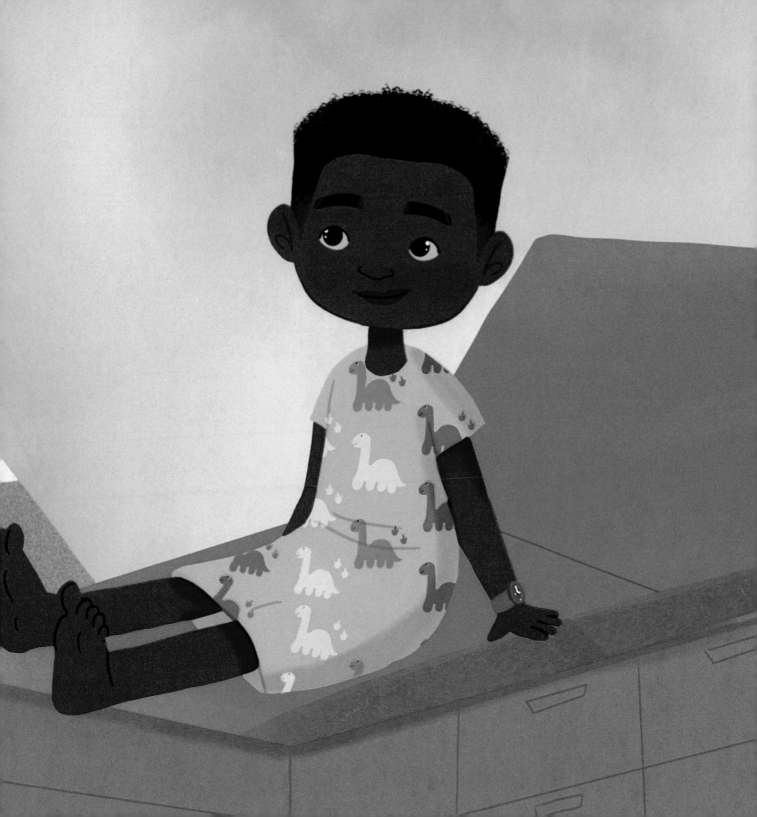

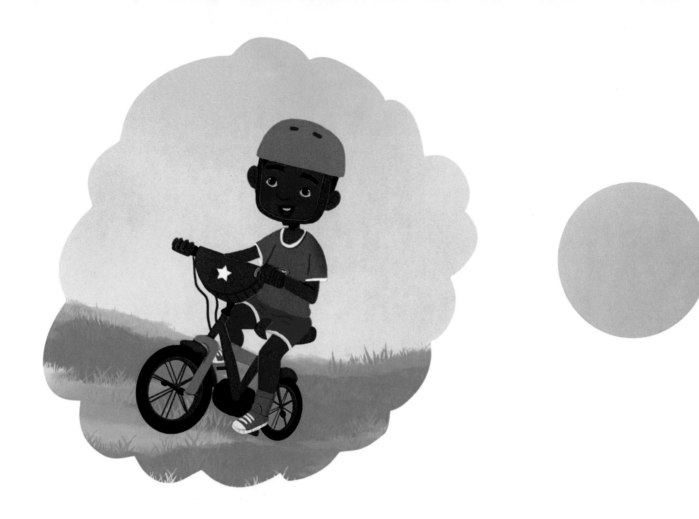

Just like when you are riding a bike,
a helmet should be on your head.

"There are other ways to keep your body safe,"
the doctor then said.

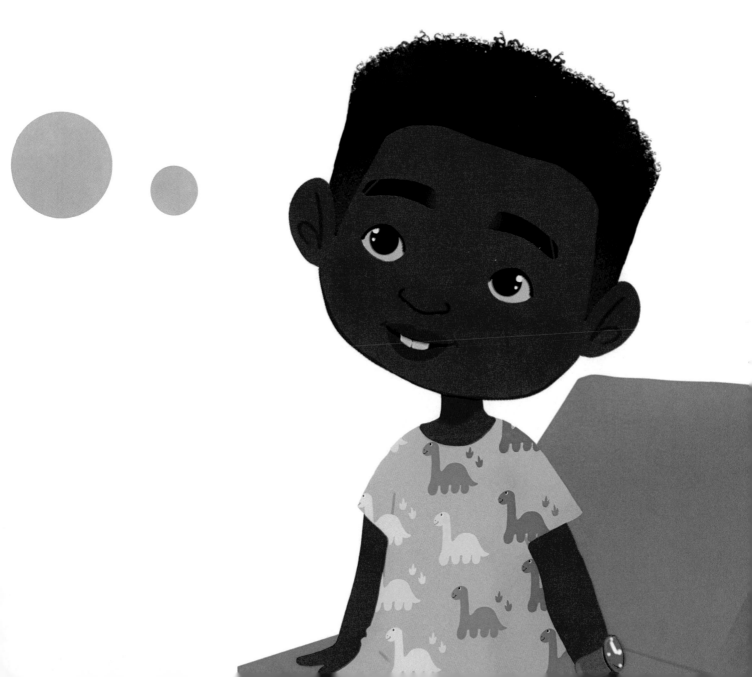

"If you're going to the pool or the beach,
what do you wear?"

"A swimsuit," I say, grinning from ear to ear.

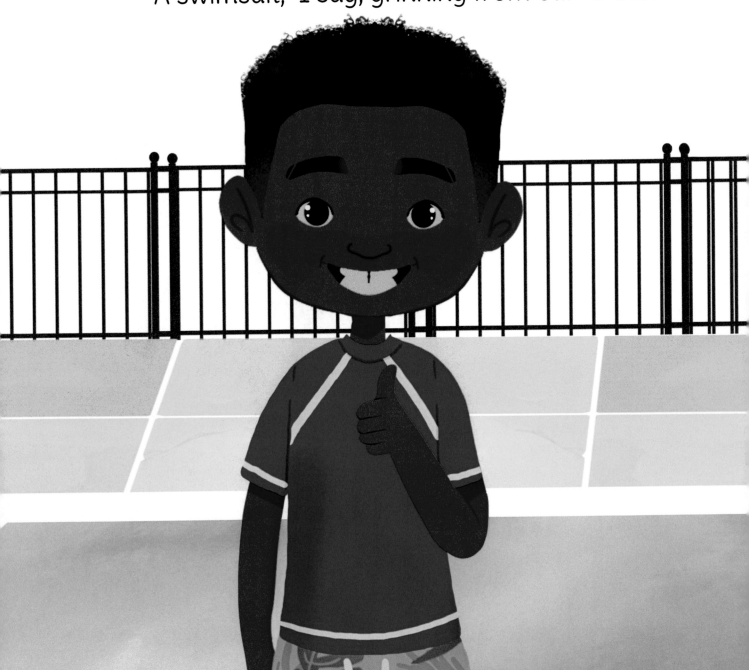

The doctor says the parts under my swimsuit
are private for me.

No one should touch there, or look there, or see.

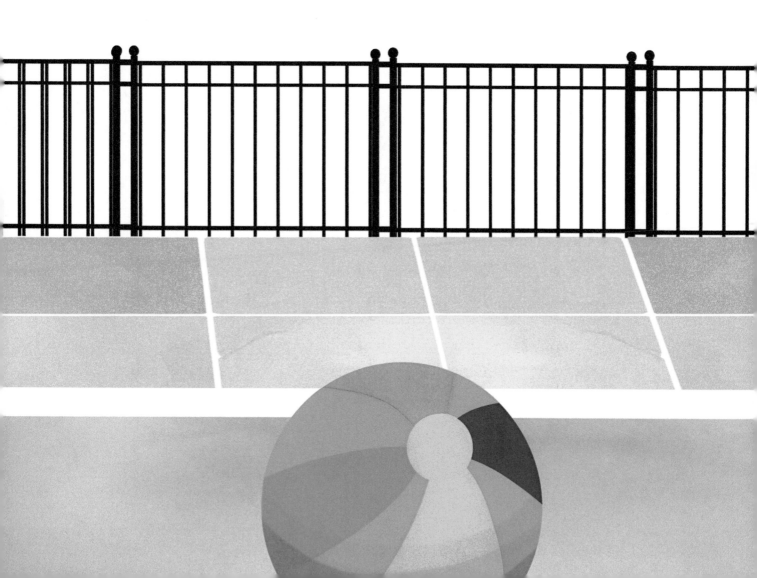

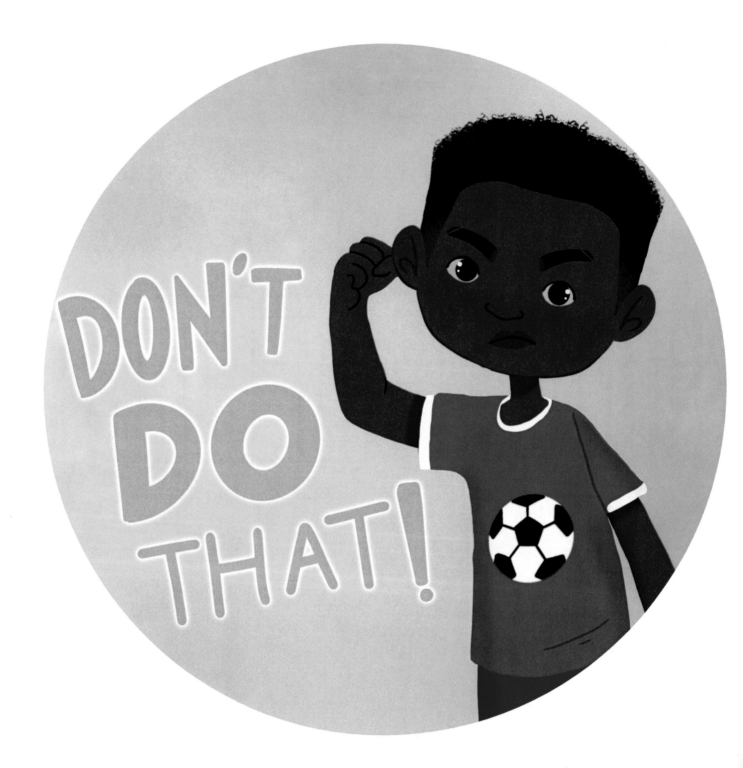

The doctor says that no one should make me do anything with my mouth.

If any of these things happen, I should say "Don't do that!" and shout!

This is my body, and I can say "NO!"

Then I must leave, be brave,
and tell a grown-up I know.

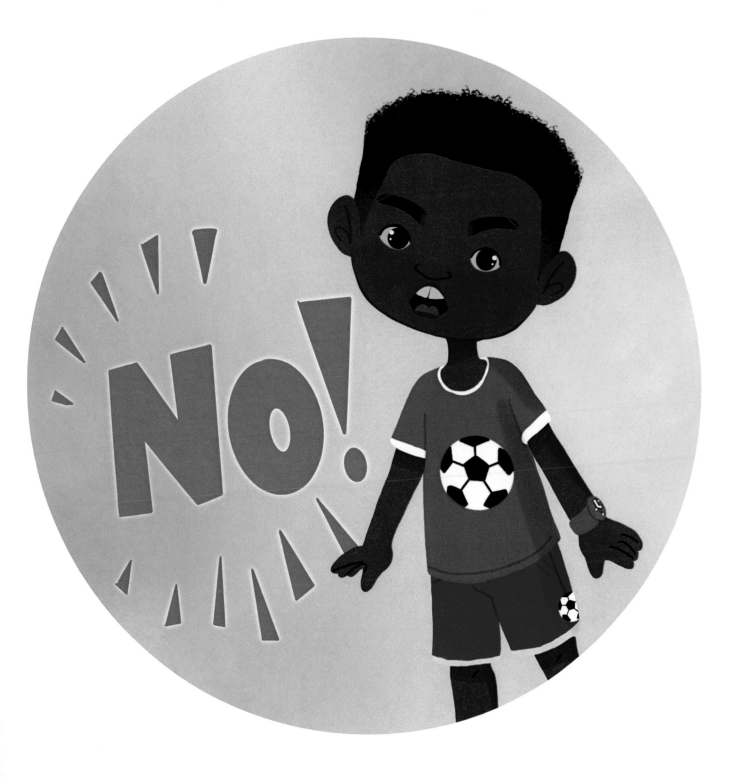

If something happens to me, I must tell right away.

There shouldn't be secrets; that's never okay.

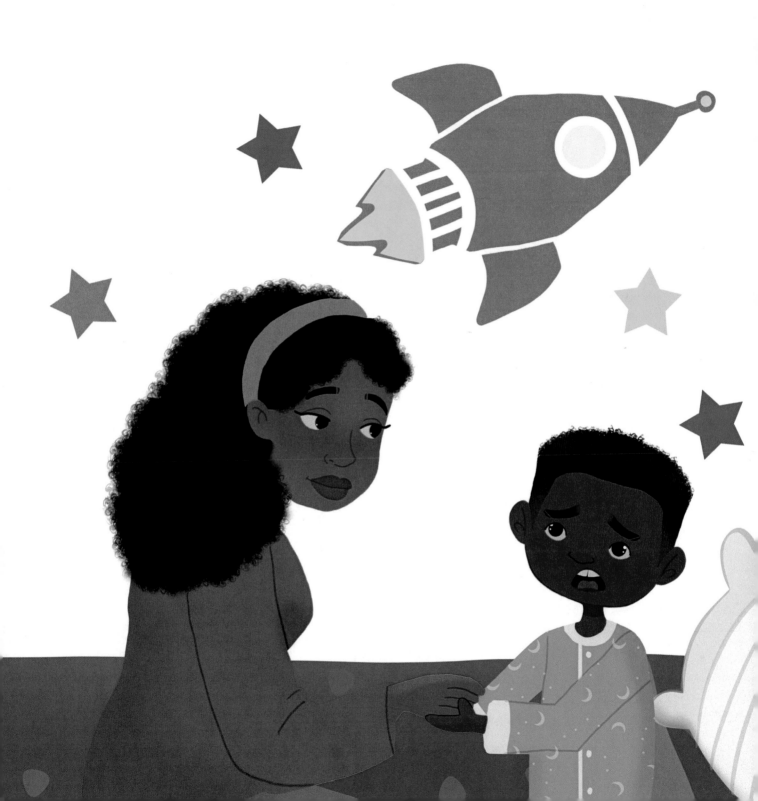

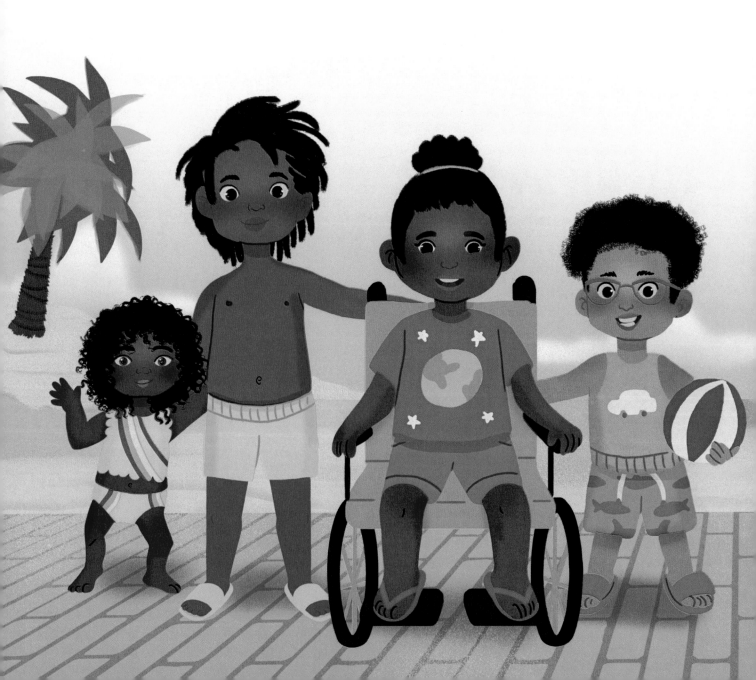

The doctor says I have rules for my body and
other kids have the same,
even if they call their private parts
by a different name.

At the end of my check-up, the doctor says,
"You're all done!"
I was brave, I listened, and we had lots of fun!

Now that I know about body safety,
I feel extra smart.
The doctor teaches me many things,
and this was just the right start!

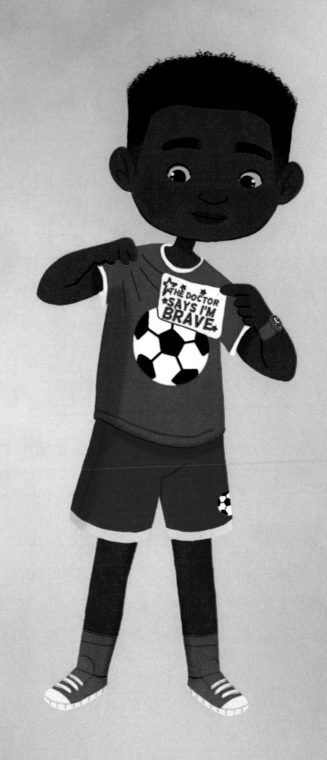

For the Grown-Ups:

AFTER you read this book with your child or have your child read this book:

It is helpful to remind your child about the most important messages. Allow your child to provide a TEACH BACK. This is a method used in health care to make sure a patient understands what was explained to them. You will ask your child to share what they have learned with you by asking them these three questions below:

a. **What are the parts of your body that no one should look at, touch, or see?**
   Answer: The parts under your swimsuit, and no one should make you do anything with your mouth.

2. **What should you do if anyone tries to do any of those things?**
   Answer: Say words like "Stop," "Don't do that," or "No" and leave. If you are too afraid to say that, you should just say that you have to leave and go somewhere safe.

3. **What should you do next if that happens?**
   Answer: Tell a grown-up right away.
   Help your child identify safe adults such as you, their grandparents, other relatives, or teacher, etc., that they could tell right away. Stress to your child that a safe grown-up will believe them.

You should speak to your child's pediatrician or pediatric health care provider for additional help. If there are immediate concerns for safety, please call 911.

For more information on this topic, please visit www.TheDoctorSays.info.

MEET THE AUTHOR

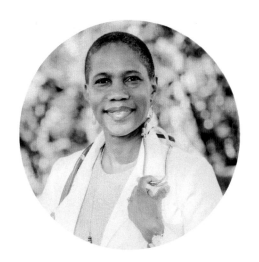

Dr. Morgan (also known as Dr. Pat) is board certified in both general pediatrics and child abuse pediatrics. From the age of eleven years old, Dr. Pat knew she wanted to be a pediatrician. She did not know that her path would lead her to care for children where there were concerns for child abuse and neglect. For over twenty years, she has shared the message of body safety during medical evaluations, and she hopes this book helps by reaching many more children and families.

MEET THE ILLUSTRATOR

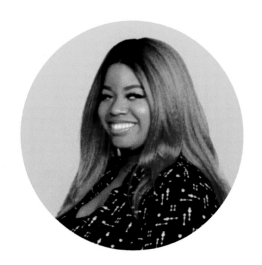

Chasity Hampton has been a professional illustrator for ten years. She started Whimsical Designs by CJ, LLC with the hope of creating art that showcases the very diverse world in which we live. Completely self-taught, she has produced original work she is proud of and collaborated with authors from around the world. She works hard to bring her clients' visions to life in her own unique style — combining traditional as well as modern illustration techniques. She hopes to continue to leave her mark (or paint) wherever she goes.

Made in United States
Orlando, FL
15 April 2023

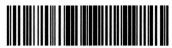
32101833R00018